UNDERSTANDING
VITAMIN-
MINERAL
SUPPLEMENTS

BY ANDREW LESSMAN

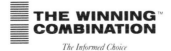

THE WINNING™
COMBINATION

The Informed Choice

Published by The Winning Combination, Inc.
1753 Cloverfield Boulevard
Santa Monica, California 90404

Designed by Don Leeds
Manufactured in the United States of America

ISBN 0-9621440-0-2

Dedicated to improving awareness.

Special thanks to Rob, David, Don, Carol, Larry,
Law and last but not least, Smithers.

CONTENTS

The Ultimate Problem:
Compromises That Lead To Unsafe & Ineffective Supplements

Currently over fifty percent of the general public and more than eighty percent of all active individuals rely on a nutritional supplement. Surprisingly, very few of these individuals realize that supplement manufacturers knowingly reduce the safety and effectiveness of their formulas by resorting to cost-cutting compromises. Fortunately, there is an alternative to these defective products.

The Only Solution:
Become An Informed Consumer

Avoiding these compromised products is as simple as learning to identify their well disguised manufacturing short-cuts and the information contained in this book is your first step in doing so. In the following pages we review and discuss the Problems brought about by the most common cost-cutting manufacturing compromises and their Solutions to seek out in the future. For ease of understanding, these Problems are divided into the four principal areas of supplement creation.

Formula Design

The first step in supplement creation concerns the most basic supplement design decisions. It involves the choice of which nutrients to include and precisely how to balance them for optimum effectiveness.

The Problem: *Poorly Balanced & Utilized Formulas*

The Solution: *Metabolic Balancing*

The most effective supplement formula is designed after considering and compensating for the impact of all metabolic processes. Such a formula is efficiently absorbed from the digestive system and rapidly taken up and utilized by your cells before it is excreted from the body.

The Facts:

It seems like a simple task to design a nutritional supplement. They appear to be nothing more than a long list of vitamins and minerals with arbitrary numbers alongside. Unfortunately, this is the same simplistic approach taken by most supplement manufacturers in the design and creation of their products. They formulate their products as if 100% of their nutrients are utilized by your body, when in reality they know that only a small percentage of the nutrients in their formulas actually succeed in being retained and used by your body.

The vitamins and minerals in a nutritional supplement are just two of the many natural components we find in food and like any food component, your body must process them prior to being used. This metabolic food processing is not 100 percent efficient and inevitably causes a reduction in the vitamins and minerals available from your supplement. In the following paragraphs we discuss the four principal metabolic processes (excluding digestion) that every nutrient encounters while in your body.

Cellular Utilization: The ultimate purpose of any supplement is to have its nutrients utilized by your cells. Utilization refers to the participation of these nutrients in cellular metabolism, such as cell growth, repair or energy production. Contrary to the approach of most manufacturers, cellular utilization of nutrients involves more than simply swallowing a tablet. Most of the nutrients in a supplement are poorly absorbed from the digestive system and even less efficiently taken up by your cells. Moreover, even if a nutrient succeeds in entering your cells, it can still freely pass back out into the bloodstream and end up being excreted without being utilized by your cells.

Your ability to utilize and benefit from a supplement means little without analyzing whether a nutrient can get to your cells in the first place. This requires consideration of the following three metabolic processes: Digestive Absorption, Cellular Uptake and Bodily Excretion. They are each discussed below.

Digestive Absorption: Before any vitamin or mineral can be utilized, it must first be extracted from food or a nutritional supplement. Ordinarily, digestion is the initiating process for absorption into the bloodstream. Fortunately, the vitamins and minerals in a supplement are in a form that does not require digestion in order for them to be absorbed into the bloodstream. The only requirement for absorption is that the vitamin-mineral tablet and its granules fully dissolve. Only after this has occurred is there any opportunity for its nutrients to enter the bloodstream.

Cellular Uptake and Bodily Excretion: Once absorbed into the bloodstream, a nutrient must quickly enter your cells or it will be promptly eliminated from the body. Our very efficient excretory system makes sure that nutrients that remain in the bloodstream are quickly removed. In other words, nutrient utilization cannot be analyzed without also considering the processes of Cellular Uptake and Bodily Excretion, since only those nutrients that survive these processes will survive to accomplish their ultimate purpose, utilization.

Every vitamin and mineral is a unique biochemical substance with its own unique chemical behavior. Once inside your body, every vitamin and mineral will exhibit different rates for each of the four metabolic processes discussed earlier. In other words, every nutrient possesses its own individual rate of Digestive Absorption, Cellular Uptake, Bodily Excretion and ultimately Utilization. When designing a formula the final concentrations of each nutrient in the product must reflect and compensate for the impact of these four metabolic processes. Unfortunately, these processes are ignored by most manufacturers.

Manufacturers continue to design formulas with label potencies that are generally nothing more than a series of rounded off arbitrary numbers or multiples of the Recommended Daily Allowances. They give no consideration to the fundamental metabolic processes that determine how well their products are utilized. The proper design requires that every nutrient in a formula be analyzed to determine its specific rates of Digestive Absorption, Cellular Uptake, Bodily Excretion and Utilization. Such a formula is referred to as being "metabolically balanced." It contains nutrients in amounts that have been carefully determined from biochemical and metabolic research. The result is a formula that does more than just deliver nutrients to your mouth. It also assures you that the proper amount and balance of these essential nutrients survive to be utilized by your cells. Any manufacturer can create an effective supplement by considering these metabolic processes in its design. Unfortunately, these features are not necessary to sell most products and therefore most manufacturers ignore them.

The Problem: *Incomplete Formulas & Non-Essential Ingredients*

The Solution: *Comprehensive Formulas With Only Essential Nutrients*

An effective vitamin-mineral supplement is made up of a complete and balanced supply of all essential vitamins and minerals along with their related co-factors and synergists. It should not contain non-essential non-vitamin, non-mineral ingredients and additives.

The Facts:

Most popular vitamin-mineral supplements include many non-vitamin, non-mineral ingredients. In general, their sole purpose for inclusion in the formula is to deceptively attract consumer interest and increase their sales. Manufacturers add trace amounts of well-publicized, non-essential ingredients such as RNA, DNA, SOD, "Vitamin B-15," Bee Pollen, Spirulina, along with numerous herbs and other non-essential components. These are just a few of the hundreds of non-vitamin, non-mineral ingredients included in most vitamin-mineral supplements. It is difficult to provide a more complete list of these popular, non-essential "nutrients" since they change so frequently.

Whether these popular "nutrients" are useful or effective is not at issue here. The experts are split on their benefits along with their potential risks. However, there is no question that these non-essential components do not belong in a vitamin-mineral formula. By introducing them in a vitamin-mineral supplement they are certain to reduce its effectiveness by impairing the absorption and uptake of its essential vitamins and minerals.

There is no reason to question a person's desire to consume these ingredients, just their judgment in consuming them as part of their vitamin-mineral supplement. Manufacturers know that adding these non-essential "nutrients" to a vitamin-mineral supplement can reduce its effectiveness. Unfortunately, these manufacturers refuse to give up an opportunity to promote new popular ingredients that will increase the sales of their vitamin-mineral supplements. Moreover, the limited space in a supplement is now taken up by non-essential ingredients that displace the essential nutrients you need.

When manufacturers place these popular, non-essential "nutrients" in a supplement, they do so in trace amounts simply to make an attractive advertising claim. The non-essential "nutrient" you seek may be present, but not in an adequate amount or form to provide any benefits. If you would like to consume this ingredient, purchase it separately from your vitamin-mineral formula, in the chemical form and amount recommended by an expert. But most importantly, do not consume it along with your vitamin-mineral supplement since doing so will only impair the effectiveness of both.

It is well-accepted that a vitamin-mineral supplement should only contain vitamins and minerals. Moreover, it should not contain just a few vitamins and minerals. It should be made up of a balanced and comprehensive blend of *all* essential vitamins and minerals. It is never prudent to employ a supplement containing a small selection of nutrients. This is because all the vitamins and minerals in your body are part of a delicate integrated balance. If you consume just one or only a few nutrients in a supplement, you run the risk of upsetting the levels of many other nutrients in your body. This is why high-dose single nutrient supplements of Calcium, Iron, Vitamin B, C and E should be used along with careful dietary planning and the support of a comprehensive and balanced vitamin-mineral supplement. This assures that your supplements play a beneficial, stabilizing role in your body rather than a disruptive, imbalancing role.

Once you have found such a supplement, it should contain metabolically balanced amounts of the following vitamins, minerals and related cofactors: Vitamins A, D, E, C (with Bioflavonoids), B-1, B-2, B-3, B-5, B-6, B-12, Folic Acid, Biotin, Choline, Inositol, PABA, Calcium, Magnesium, Manganese, Molybdenum, Copper, Iron, Zinc, Selenium, Chromium, Phosphorus, Iodine, Boron, Cobalt, Vanadium and Germanium. For additional information on which chemical forms and sources of these nutrients to seek out, read on.

The Problem: *Acid Induced Nutrient Damage & Stomach Discomfort*

The Solution: *Buffering, Stabilizing & Balancing pH*

An effective supplement formula is designed to prevent the nutrient destruction, reduced absorption and stomach discomfort caused by the extremes of digestive pH. This is readily accomplished by a careful balance of nutrients that stabilize and buffer the pH.

The Facts:

The digestion of food requires an extremely acidic environment, while the subsequent absorption of its constituent nutrients requires an extremely alkaline environment. These normal extremes of digestive acidity and alkalinity can result in severe damage to the vitamins and minerals in your nutritional supplement.

Scientists refer to the relative acidity or alkalinity of any system according to an accepted measuring system referred to as the pH scale. The pH scale begins at 1 and increases to a maximum reading of 14. A pH of 1 corresponds to the most acidic pH possible, while at the other end of the scale a pH of 14 corresponds to the most basic or alkaline pH possible. The mid-point of the pH scale is at 7 and corresponds to the totally neutral pH of pure water.

The stomach is one of the most acidic environments possible. It is hard to believe that its contents exist at a pH between 1 and 2. This acidity is so extreme that it would eat its way out of virtually any man-made container. Fortunately, it is confined and protected by the mucosal lining of the stomach. This extreme acidity is vital for the digestion of food but can also damage the delicate vitamins and minerals in most nutritional supplements. This damage is brought about by a myriad of chemical reactions that destroy your valuable nutrients.

Immediately following the extreme acidity of the stomach is the highly alkaline environment of the small intestine. This is where virtually all nutrient absorption takes place. It is therefore vitally important that as many nutrients as possible survive the extreme pH of the stomach and move on to the small intestine. Moreover, when they arrive in the small intestine, they must exist in a usable, absorbable form.

All in all, the digestive system presents a very hostile environment to the delicate contents of a nutritional supplement. It is up to the manufacturer to design and balance a formula that remains optimally effective in the face of this pH-induced nutrient damage. In doing so, the manufacturer will also eliminate the stomach discomfort that accompanies the use of poorly balanced ordinary formulas. This is accomplished by choosing vitamins and minerals that can perform as active buffers at extreme digestive pH. In other words, a manufacturer must look at the pH characteristics of each and every nutrient, not just as an individual, but as a part of the total formula. Unfortunately, very few manufacturers take these steps.

The Problem: *Adverse Competition & Interactions Among Nutrients*

The Solution: *Balanced Non-Competitive, Non-Interactive Formulas*
The most effective supplement is designed using a balance of ingredients that prevents nutrient competition or adverse ingredient interactions. Multiple ingredient combinations are tested and analyzed in order to arrive at a formula with the smallest probability of destructive ingredient interactions and competition.

The Facts:
Most nutritional supplements contain a large assortment of vitamins and minerals. In most cases, a comprehensive supplement will contain between 25 and 40 different nutrients. These vitamins and minerals do not only participate in beneficial chemical reactions in your body, they will also engage in many less desirable chemical reactions. This occurs when the dozens of vitamins and

minerals present in a supplement arrive simultaneously in your digestive system. They chemically interact as a result of their inherent chemical properties which are further aggravated by the extreme acidity of the stomach.

The supplement eventually leaves the stomach and next moves on to the very alkaline environment of the small intestine. For a nutritional supplement, this is the most critical portion of the digestive system because it is where virtually all nutrient absorption occurs. Unfortunately, this absorption does not take place unobstructed. Many chemical reactions continue between nutrients as a result of the alkaline pH of the small intestine. Making matters even worse is the "competition" for absorption between various nutrients. Some nutrients "win" and are absorbed; others "lose" and pass through your body unutilized. The real loser is you, when nutrients compete and are excreted, unused.

Nutrient competition can be prevented in much the same way that pH damage and stomach discomfort are avoided. It simply requires an analysis of the various nutrients in the supplement and their potential to either chemically interact with each other or to compete for absorption. The potential interactions and competition can be corrected by balancing the pH of the formula and employing chemical forms of the nutrients that have a lesser tendency toward these adverse interactions. A manufacturer must build this into the original design of the supplement long before it is produced. Unfortunately the expense of planning for and avoiding these problems discourages manufacturers from taking these steps.

Ingredient Selection

The second step in supplement creation concerns the selection of each of the specific nutrients to be included in the formula. It involves the choice of the chemical form, source, quality and purity of each vitamin and mineral included in the product.

The Problem: *Deceptive Use Of Low Activity Nutrients*

The Solution: *Maximum Bioactivity Ingredients*

A highly effective supplement formula must contain the most bioactive molecular form of each ingredient. Such a design must contain more than a token amount of the most efficiently absorbed and utilized chemical forms of each nutrient.

The Facts:

Every vitamin and mineral exists naturally in hundreds of chemical forms. For example, Vitamin C exists naturally as Ascorbic Acid, Calcium Ascorbate, Potassium Ascorbate and Ascorbyl Palmitate to name just four. Although each is still Vitamin C, they all possess very different chemical and molecular structures. It is these molecular variations that account for the dramatic differences in chemical properties between various chemical forms of the same nutrient. Bioactivity is perhaps the most important of these chemical properties, since it is a direct measure of the ability of a particular nutrient to benefit you.

Following years of testing, researchers have determined the most bioactive and desirable molecular forms in which to deliver most vitamins. They have also determined the less active forms to avoid. With regard to a few key vitamins, the most bioactive and readily utilized forms are as follows:

Vitamin C *in the form of Calcium Ascorbate and Ascorbyl Palmitate rather than ordinary Ascorbic Acid.*

Vitamin A *in the form of Natural Beta Carotene.*

Vitamin B-2 *in the form of Riboflavin-5-Phosphate rather than only Riboflavin.*

Vitamin B-3 *in the form of Niacin rather than only Niacinamide.*

Vitamin B-6 *in the form of Pyridoxyl-5-Phosphate rather than only Pyridoxine.*

Vitamin E *in the form of oil-free d-Alpha Tocopherol Succinate.*

As for minerals, the research indicates that they are generally most bioactive when consumed in the form of a true amino acid-mineral chelate. A "true amino acid chelate" is a chemical combination of an individual mineral linked to a specific amino acid. There are just over 20 naturally occurring amino acids and only a select few of these are chemically capable of binding with a mineral to form such chelates. Moreover, there is a specific amino acid that is the ideal partner for each mineral and results in a significant increase in its bioactivity. This increase in bioactivity results from that amino acid acting as a more efficient transporter of the mineral, thereby enhancing its absorption, uptake and utilization.

A true amino acid chelate is the result of a specially designed and controlled reaction between a pure quantity of a mineral with a pure supply of its appropriate amino acid partner. The resulting pure amino acid mineral chelate possesses new, more desirable properties that neither the individual amino acid nor the mineral alone possessed previously.

Unfortunately, most manufacturers do not employ true amino acid chelates. They employ low cost, "counterfeit" amino acid mineral chelates. These counterfeit chelates are made by enzymatically digesting protein in the presence of extreme acids and caustic alkaline chemicals. They result in nothing more than a toxic and contaminated concoction of partially digested protein with damaged amino acids.

After adding minerals to this concoction, manufacturers refer to them as amino acid mineral chelates or proteinates. These mineral concoctions possess none of the desirable properties of a true amino mineral chelate. They are easy to spot since the formula's label never states the name of a specific amino acid. It may only state general language such as "amino acid chelate or proteinate." They cannot provide the name of a specific amino acid because it is actually made from digested protein with its twenty amino acids, rather than a single pure amino acid. The only assurance that you are getting a true amino acid chelate is when the name of the individual amino acid is specified.

Certain amino acids possess properties that enable them to act as very efficient transporters of various minerals. Aspartic Acid is an amino acid that acts as an excellent transporter for Calcium, Magnesium, Manganese, Zinc, Molybdenum, Potassium and Boron. Its biochemical properties enable it to enhance the ability of these minerals to be absorbed and utilized by your cells. Fully reacted chelates of each of these minerals with Aspartic Acid are referred to as Aspartates and are the preferred form of delivering these minerals. Three other minerals, Chromium, Iron and Cobalt are most bioactive when bound to the amino acid Glycine and are referred to as Glycinates. Selenium on the other hand is most active when bound to Methionine to form Selenomethionine. It is vitally important that the name of the specific amino acid, such as an Aspartate, Glycinate or Methionine appear on the label. General words such as "amino acid chelate" or "proteinate" should immediately steer you away from that product since it is probably not a genuine chelate. Moreover, the actual amino acid's name is your only means of determining if the chelate in question is the most active form available, such as an Aspartate or Glycinate.

Another deceptive sales tactic employed by manufacturers is the use of "misleading label claims." The most desirable and expensive forms of the vitamins and minerals discussed previously are the subject of these deceptive marketing practices. They appear on hundreds of labels, yet mysteriously make up only a minute percentage of the formulas. Instead, virtually all the vitamins and minerals in most supplements are included in a less expensive and less desirable form. When expensive nutrients do appear, it is generally only in trace amounts to enable an attractive but misleading label claim.

The Problem: *Synthetic Nutrients Derived From Petroleum*

The Solution: *Nutrients Derived From All Natural Sources*

Natural source ingredients which do not contain synthetically produced contaminants and also possess naturally occurring co-factors, synergists and molecular structures that enhance their activity and effectiveness.

The Facts:

It's hard to believe, but most of the vitamins present in conventional supplements are chemically produced from petroleum. This is the same petroleum that is used to fuel your car. Who would think that crude oil would be used to produce the vitamins we rely upon as well? Although common to most products, these synthetic nutrients are far from desirable. They can include toxic residues remaining from their manufacture and also lack the co-factors and synergists that accompany and enhance the activity of natural nutrients. The low cost of these mass produced artificial nutrients is the reason for their abundance in ordinary supplements.

A very common but unique property of vitamins gives rise to an unusual problem with synthetic vitamins. The problem stems from the unique three dimensional structure that each vitamin possesses. This isn't a problem until the vitamin attempts to take part in your body's chemical reactions. A simple illustration will make it more clear. All of your body's chemical reactions and processes are dependent upon the work of vitamins and enzymes. These vital substances function by fitting themselves together into a very rigorously organized structure in the body. When all the components are perfectly oriented and arranged, the appropriate chemical reactions can take place. Unless they are perfectly arranged, none of these chemical reactions can occur. Herein lies the problem with many synthetic nutrients.

The easiest way to look at the problem is to imagine the way a hand and glove interrelate. If a glove is the proper size and has the correct number of fingers, then it should fit. But it isn't that simple. The glove for your right hand will not fit your left hand and vice versa. Even though your left and right glove or hand are the exact same size and possess the same number of fingers, the gloves will never be interchangeable. This is because even though your hands appear the same, technically, they are not. They are actually mirror images of each other and although they appear identical, they cannot wear the same glove.

It is precisely the same with vitamins. Synthetic vitamins are often the exact mirror image of their natural counterparts. Unfortunately, your body's biochemistry is either right or left handed, but never both. Your body is equipped to recognize and use only the naturally occurring form of the vitamin and not its synthetic mirror image counterpart. It would be like trying to put a left-handed glove on your right hand. It just won't work. Moreover, in the case of some nutrients like Carnitine, the synthetic counterpart is not only inactive, it is also toxic.

In the final analysis, there is little reason to consume a synthetically produced supplement. They are potentially toxic, contaminated and often inactive. With the ready availability of natural source nutrients it would seem foolish to second guess mother nature. The logical solution is a natural source supplement. Unfortunately, a true natural supplement is both difficult to locate and unless selected carefully can often be far from perfect.

The Problem: *Highly Allergic Nutrient Sources*

The Solution: *Supplements Free Of All Common Allergens*
The safest and most effective formulas avoid nutrient sources that contain any allergens and instead employ completely hypo-allergenic nutrient sources. Such formulas must also be free of additives or synthetic ingredients, which are a proven source of additional allergens.

The Facts:
It has long been established that any food or chemical can cause an allergic reaction. Naturally, it makes sense to avoid exposure to any potentially allergic foods or substances. Unfortunately, most supplement manufacturers deprive consumers of their ability to avoid these potentially allergic ingredients. They include many nutrients in forms derived from the most allergenic food sources. Making matters worse is the fact that these food sources are concentrated for use in a supplement which only serves to further concentrate the allergens they contain.

To cut costs, most manufacturers choose their ingredients from highly allergic foods. Not surprisingly, allergic reactions from nutritional supplements are growing more and more common. These allergic reactions aren't the sneezing, wheezing, hives and rashes we ordinarily associate with hay fever or other allergies. Instead, they are the subtle symptoms that are more characteristic of ordinary food allergies. Supplement allergies most frequently result in unexplained headaches, drowsiness, water retention, irritability, depression and most often fatigue. Avoiding these allergic reactions is as simple as avoiding allergenic supplement ingredients.

Each nutrient in a supplement formula can be obtained from thousands of natural food sources. Like any food, these nutrient sources can cause allergic reactions. Moreover, by concentrating a nutrient source for use in a supplement, the allergens they may contain also become more concentrated. The most common sources of Vitamin C (corn), Vitamin A (fish oil), Vitamin D (fish oil), Vitamin E (soy), most B vitamins (wheat and other grains) and chelates (milk and egg derivatives) are medically accepted as highly allergic. Nevertheless, these allergic foods continue to be the most common source for all of these nutrients. It is the low cost of these harmful nutrient sources that encourages manufacturers to overlook their common allergens and to continue using them in their formulas.

When purchasing a supplement, it makes sense to avoid allergenic ingredients such as corn, milk, yeast, wheat, liver, soy and fish oils. Unfortunately, it is difficult to determine the source of most of the nutrients in a supplement because most manufacturers do not provide that information on their labels. Generally, when a claim is not made to the contrary, a manufacturer employs a synthetic form or the least expensive natural form with its abundance of common allergens.

The use of highly allergic ingredients isn't something to be taken lightly. The subtle yet cumulative harm that can result from daily consumption of these allergens can be particularly troublesome. These allergies can have a significant impact on the quality of your health and life. Often, it is very easy to become accustomed to these subtle allergic reactions without ever discerning their cause. It isn't until an aware physician takes notice or simply by accident that the cause can be established and eliminated.

Allergic reactions are also caused by the contaminants and impurities that accompany any low quality supplement, whether natural or synthetic. Chemical additives offer the worst of both worlds. These binders, fillers, lubricants, flowing agents and excipients can be either synthetically or naturally derived. This means that they can carry the impurities and contaminants of their synthetic manufacture or high concentrations of allergens from their natural source.

Since they aren't active ingredients, it is easy to overlook the allergic potential of these chemical additives even though they comprise between ten and sixty percent of all supplements. In light of this, even if a supplement's nutrients are completely hypo-allergenic, it is of little consequence unless the chemical additives it contains are also hypo-allergenic.

The Problem: *Low Quality Contaminated Ingredients*

The Solution: *Optimally Pure Contaminant-Free Nutrients*
    Safety is assured by using the highest quality ingredients to meet the highest standards for purity. This is achieved by avoiding all chemical additives and maintaining continuous laboratory testing of all nutrients to ensure the absence of unsuspected contamination.

The Facts:
    Every ingredient in a supplement is available in a wide range of purities. This range begins at almost 100 percent purity and ends at the rather low levels of purity common to most popular supplements. These lower levels of purity are referred to as food grade purity. It is best characterized by the fruits and vegetables in the produce aisle of your supermarket. Despite a relatively high content of impurities, these foods are acceptable for sale. The Food and Drug Administration gives markets a great deal of latitude in this regard. That is why we carefully select our food at the market and then we scrub, rinse and peel our food before we eat it at home. Unfortunately, we can't do the same to our nutritional supplements.
    With regard to purity, vitamins and minerals are considered to be no more than foods. Therefore, they must only meet the very lax purity standards established for all ordinary foods. These relatively impure formulas do not violate any laws and are indicative of the industry standard for purity. Oddly enough, a vitamin supplement doesn't have to be as pure as an over-the-counter medication. In other words, the drugs you periodically must consume for an illness are usually purer than the supplement you consume every day for your health.
    Most popular supplement formulas are made with low-cost, impure ingredients. They contain known contaminated nutrient sources, such as dolomite, bone meal, oyster shell, egg shell, fish oils, sea sediment, beef or fish livers, etc. These common nutrient sources have been found to contain organic contaminants and toxic heavy metals including lead, arsenic, cadmium, aluminum and nickel. They grow, live and die in our oceans or other parts of our polluted environment. They also contain residues of pesticides, hormones, antibiotics and other harmful organic chemicals. For example, the fish that swim in our polluted oceans depend upon their livers to filter out this pollution. Incredibly,

contaminated fish livers are the most common source of Vitamin A and D. Similarly, oysters that reside on our polluted coastline concentrate more than just Calcium in their shells. Once again, these contaminated shells are the most common source of Calcium in the form of Calcium Carbonate. Concentrating these nutrient sources for use in a supplement makes the contaminants they contain even more potent and dangerous. The list of these common contaminated nutrient sources is shocking; but unfortunately, their extremely low cost, continues to encourage manufacturers to overlook their risks.

The purity of a supplement's nutrients aren't the only point of concern. It is also important to be aware of the presence of any chemical additives in the formula, since these additives generally do not meet the same purity requirements as the supplement's nutrients. This is of particular concern because most vitamin-mineral supplements contain larger amounts of these additives than they do any other single nutrient.

In order to create supplements at the highest levels of purity, a manufacturer must perform ongoing laboratory tests of all raw materials and ingredients. Unfortunately, since this is not legally required and is also quite expensive, few manufacturers do so. Not surprisingly, the result is that the FDA frequently impounds product that fails to meet even the most minimal of purity standards. The abuses are so common that even with their limited resources, the FDA still manages to catch numerous violations. Unfortunately, the FDA's budget does not permit frequent inspection of many nutritional supplements, so you can't rely on them to protect the purity of your formula. Your only assurance of purity is to purchase a formula that is independently laboratory tested and constantly monitored by its manufacturer.

The Problem: *High Levels Of Toxic Nutrients*

The Solution: *Absolutely Non-Toxic Amounts and Forms of Nutrients*

The safest formula avoids any ingredient that can potentially build-up to toxic levels in the body. This requires the use of the safest molecular form and careful consideration of the amount of each nutrient present in a formula.

The Facts:

It shocks most consumers when they discover that the nutrients present in most supplements are potentially toxic. Supplements are supposed to be healthful, not harmful. Unfortunately, many nutrients employed in ordinary supplements are present in chemical forms and amounts that can be toxic. Toxicity results when a specific nutrient builds up in the body. This occurs when a supplement includes too much of a nutrient or employs it in a chemical form that is poorly excreted from the body. The result is a gradual accumulation of this nutrient which will eventually become toxic.

Manufacturers take no steps to eliminate these inexpensive, yet toxic nutrients from their formulas. On the contrary, unscrupulous manufacturers take advantage of unaware consumers who assume that if 100 milligrams works well, then 1,000 milligrams works better. Manufacturers continue to make formulas with escalating doses of inexpensive toxic nutrients. Consumers unknowingly abuse these formulas and expose themselves to unnecessary toxic risks. Making matters worse is the fact that many of the formulas with the highest nutrient levels are also the products that contain the most toxic forms of those nutrients.

The most glaring and well documented examples of toxic reactions from accumulated high doses of vitamins have occurred with Vitamins A, D and B-6. There are numerous safe alternatives to the chemical forms and amounts that gave rise to these toxic reactions. For example, Beta Carotene is an absolutely non-toxic form of Vitamin A. Similarly, since Vitamin D is readily produced when the skin is exposed to sunlight, there is no need to include a large amount of it in any supplement. Similarly, toxicity from Vitamin B-6 is readily eliminated by adjusting its chemical form and amount.

Toxic reactions have also been observed with certain minerals such as Selenium, Chromium, Iron, Molybdenum and Copper. Specifically, the non-chelated forms of these minerals can be very toxic and dangerous even when consumed at relatively low levels. Accordingly, safer chemical forms of these minerals, generally in the form of chelates should be employed to eliminate these problems.

An ethical manufacturer must recognize and plan for the natural human tendency to sometimes consume more than the recommended dose of a product. Under such circumstances, it is the responsibility of the manufacturer to choose chemical forms that reduce or eliminate any toxic risks. Unfortunately, most manufacturers look the other way and refuse to invest the additional money to purchase costly, but safe non-toxic nutrients. In fact many go to the other extreme and continue to play "a numbers game," steadily increasing the numbers on the label.

Formula Production

This third step in supplement creation concerns the production of the nutritional supplement. It involves decisions that effect the physical production and biochemistry of the manufacturing process.

The Problem: *Nutrients Damaged & Destroyed By Heat*

The Solution: *Entirely Cold Processed Formulas*

The most effective supplement is never subjected to the damaging effects of heat. This absolutely precludes the use of heat-generating processes, such as tableting or friction-grinding in the preparation of an effective supplement.

The Facts:

Heat is the single most damaging environmental condition that a supplement's ingredients can be exposed to during manufacture. High temperatures encourage oxidation (reactions with oxygen), hydrolysis (reactions with water) and even chemical reactions among the nutrients themselves. The net result of these chemical changes is a significant, if not total loss of the product's activity. Surprisingly, it isn't external heat that causes this damage, but heat generated by the manufacturing process itself.

In order to expedite and facilitate manufacturing, the ingredients in most supplements are ground into a suitable granular form. These coarse granules flow more easily throughout production and can be more easily compressed into a tablet. At first glance, conventional granulation may seem beneficial because it produces a finer, more readily dissolved powder. Unfortunately, the process of granulating these nutrients is performed by friction-grinding which produces high levels of heat. The heat generated in grinding supplements is so severe that it can actually melt the ingredients themselves. These ground-up nutrients are then heated once again, when they are crushed under several tons of pressure to form a tablet. This heat results from the rapid and dramatic increase in pressure that is an inevitable part of the tableting process. The nutrients in all tablets are damaged or destroyed by the heat that results from being crushed under twenty to fifty thousand pounds of pressure. Just as overcooking destroys the nutrients in food, the extreme heat of grinding and tableting destroys the nutritional value of most supplements.

Products in capsules are created without the pressure and resulting heat caused by tableting. Similarly, there are numerous methods of granulating ingredients without exposing them to friction and its accompanying heat. Unfortunately, the solutions to these problems cost more than most manufacturers are willing to invest in their products. It should therefore come as no surprise that cold processed encapsulated formulas are never easy to locate.

The Problem: *Insoluble, Inactive & Ineffective Supplements*

The Solution: *Rapidly Absorbed Ultra-fine Powders In Capsules*

The most rapidly absorbed formulas are microgranulated into ultra-fine granules that dissolve instantly. They are then placed in a capsule that immediately releases its contents for absorption. Moreover, encapsulation avoids the harmful heat and additives of the tableting process.

The Facts:

Nutrients cannot be absorbed from your digestive tract unless they first dissolve. Just as powdered sugar dissolves faster than a sugar cube, a finely powdered formula in a capsule dissolves far quicker than the same formula in a tablet. The powder dissolves quickly because of the cumulative surface area of its millions of tiny granules that are exposed to the digestive fluids. On the other hand, a tablet has a relatively small surface area exposed to digestive fluids and it is also usually smooth, hard and impermeable. The end result is that the fine grains in a capsule dissolve and are immediately available for absorption, while a tablet dissolves poorly, often passing through the digestive system entirely intact.

Your digestive system is composed of several organs, including the mouth, esophagus, stomach, small intestine and large intestine. Virtually no nutrient absorption occurs in the stomach or large intestine. On the other hand, almost all nutrient absorption occurs in the very first part of the small intestine referred to as the duodenum and jejunum, which immediately follows the stomach. This critical absorptive area is responsible for over 90% of all nutrient absorption. Ordinarily, a supplement is beyond this small absorptive area within a few hours of being consumed. If a supplement tablet has not fully dissolved by the time it leaves your stomach and enters this area, then no absorption can take place. In other words, a tablet's large, insoluble, coated granules generally lack sufficient time to dissolve and therefore pass through the digestive system unabsorbed and unused.

This same line of reasoning invalidates the hype and claims surrounding time release products. You don't need to read the detailed medical studies to understand why time release products are nothing more than fraudulent claims. It is medically accepted that any supplement is long past the only absorptive site in your body within a few hours of consumption. This means that absorption ceases within a few hours of swallowing the tablet. How then could a tablet continue to be absorbed into your system for 8, 12 or even 24 hours? By then the tablet has already left your body. It may continue to time-release for 8, 12 or even 24 hours, but without any benefit to you, since it is no longer in your body!

You may have noticed that many vitamin-mineral tablets are a familiar shade of brown. This is unusual since most vitamins and minerals occur naturally as a pale shade of white or yellow. This means that the manufacturer has added materials to the product to result in this brown color. Aside from a manufacturer's general tendency to abuse unnecessary additives, there would seem to be no purpose for coloring a supplement this familiar shade of brown. However, when you consider the possibility of a tablet not dissolving in your digestive system and exiting your body visibly intact, the reason for this familiar color becomes clear.

The Problem: *Abuse of Harmful Chemical Additives*

The Solution: *Formulas With Absolutely No Additives*

Additive-free products are far safer and more effective than their additive laden counterparts. Additive-free products are generally found in capsules and will specifically state that they "contain only the active ingredients named on the label and no additives of any kind."

The Facts:

Virtually every nutritional supplement is loaded with undesirable chemical additives. They are necessary to make supplement production an efficient and inexpensive process. Unfortunately, vitamins and minerals do not naturally stick together when compressed in a tableting machine. Because of their highly crystalline structure, they fall apart during the tableting process. As a result, manufacturers must employ large amounts of glue-like additives to improve the efficiency of the tableting process. These additives make the nutrient granules readily stick to each other when compressed in a tableting press. They are referred to as binders and work best when they uniformly coat all the vitamin and mineral granules in a supplement.

The "clumpy," crystalline properties of vitamins and minerals, plus the high concentrations of glue-like binders create a need for further additives. A manufacturer must include additives that lubricate and speed the flow of ingredients into the tableting mold or capsuling machine, without counteracting the effect of the binders. These additives are generally referred to as lubricants, flowing agents or excipients and are found in virtually every supplement product made.

Unlike binders and lubricants, the last group of chemical additives do not play a role in making the manufacturing process faster or more efficient. They are additives that are employed to mislead the consumer by producing a product that appears more appealing. For example, in order for a tablet or a capsule to appear full when completed, manufacturers use fluffy additives called fillers. Tablets are coated with glazes, artificial colors and flavors to enhance their appearance and taste. As discussed above, artificial colors can also be employed to disguise a supplement's departure from your body.

Additives make manufacturing faster and less expensive. Unfortunately, they also make supplements harmful and for the most part insoluble and useless. Binders make the nutrients in these rock-hard glued together tablets stick together so well that they cannot dissolve in your stomach. Lubricants, excipients and other additives only serve to further impair the absorption of any supplement. Perhaps the worst thought of all is that eventually all of these unwanted and potentially harmful chemical additives must be processed and hopefully excreted by your body.

A capsule is unquestionably superior to a tablet because it dissolves quickly, and is made without the heat and binders of tableting. Unfortunately, even manufacturers that make encapsulated products are now using additives to reduce the cost of the encapsulation process. These additives are as undesirable as those in any tablet. They generally take the form of flowing agents and lubricants to facilitate the flow of nutrients throughout the manufacturing process and insure that the capsule will seal without breakage. Manufacturers also employ fillers in order to make the capsules "appear" completely and equally full. These inexpensive, mass produced, additive-laden capsules are not much better than the tablets they were intended to replace.

Product Protection

The fourth and last phase in supplement creation concerns the steps that must be taken to insure optimum product safety and effectiveness. It involves decisions that relate to the continued development of the product, along with its overall production, packaging, marketing and distribution.

The Problem: *Outdated & Obsolete Supplements*

The Solution: *Continuous Product Research, Development & Updating*

To maintain optimum safety and effectiveness a formula must be constantly updated to include the most recent developments in medical research and manufacturing technology. The safest and most effective formulas have been updated to include most or all of the developments described in this book.

The Facts:

Every year, thousands of research studies are concluded containing important information relevant to the design and manufacture of nutritional supplements. To a few concerned and quality-oriented manufacturers, these studies are the key to improving the safety and effectiveness of their supplement formulas. Unfortunately, to the overwhelming majority of supplement manufacturers, these studies are nothing more than something to overlook or ignore. It isn't that they are not interested in these advances and improvements, it is simply that they need not spend money on product development when their existing formulas are selling so well. The research has established that for each of the problems discussed in this booklet, there is a readily available solution. These solutions are not a trade secret or mystery. The only mystery is why companies rarely update their products by instituting them.

The information contained in this book is the same information that manufacturers have ignored for decades. For instance, research relating to metabolic and pH balancing, more pure and active nutrients, less allergenic and toxic ingredients, along with advanced production and packaging technology have all been the subject of numerous studies. Unfortunately, all of these improvements and advances are more expensive than the older methods that have been around for decades. The increased expense that is involved with updating and upgrading these antique formulas has preserved them essentially unchanged for years. All in all, supplement manufacturers loyalty to profits has prevented them from providing you with the benefits of thirty years of progress. As long as consumers continue to buy the same defective products they did thirty years ago, there will be little reason for manufacturers to institute these changes.

The Problem: *Protracted Production Delays*

The Solution: *Uninterrupted, One-Step Manufacturing*

To maintain optimum safety and potency, a supplement must be manufactured in one continuous process with no interruptions or delays between production steps, all the way through to packaging. By rapidly producing and sealing a product in its protective packaging, a manufacturer decreases the chance of damage during the most vulnerable stages of production.

The Facts:

Most popular supplements require months to progress from raw materials to finished product. A supplement begins as raw materials stored in the warehouse of a major chemical supplier. These materials are then shipped to the supplement manufacturer and usually reside there for days, months or even years before they are eventually used. During these delays, the storage containers for these raw materials can be frequently opened for use in the production of other products. This is quite common since most manufacturers produce dozens, if not hundreds of other formulas. Most of these formulas have several common ingredients, particularly the manufacturing additives such as binders and lubricants that are used in each of them. As a result, most manufacturers maintain a warehouse containing large quantities of common ingredients that are repeatedly sealed and unsealed and exposed to purity and potency robbing factors.

In most facilities, these ingredients do not immediately complete the production process, but must wait their turn to be blended, granulated, dried, tableted or encapsulated. Once all of the ingredients are assembled, they are blended together to initiate the production process. They can wait months or more to complete production. During these delays, they continue to run the risk of being exposed to potency robbing factors. Finally, the process is completed when the supplement is packaged. Unfortunately, these packaging materials rarely offer adequate protection against further product deterioration.

These long unprotected delays are characteristic of the minor role that quality-control plays in the production decisions made by most manufacturers. It is during these delays between the numerous stages of manufacture and packaging that a formula is at greatest risk of exposure to harmful environmental factors. The longer it takes for a supplement to progress from raw materials to a packaged product, the greater the likelihood of damage while in a raw and vulnerable form. Unfortunately, most manufacturing facilities are neither temperature nor humidity controlled and by the time the product reaches you, its potency is a fraction of what it was intended to be.

The Problem: *Inadequate & Unprotective Packaging*

The Solution: *Multiple Barrier Protective Packaging*

The effectiveness of a high bioactivity supplement can only be maintained by protecting it from the destructive effects of air, moisture, heat, light and aging. Recent advances in multi-layered packeting materials allow the creation of a virtual 100% barrier to these damaging environmental factors.

The Facts:

A supplement that has endured the damage brought about by long un-protected delays in the production process is no better off once it is placed in its final packaging. No matter how effective a supplement is when it is produced, its effectiveness can only be maintained if it is protected from the destructive effects of air, moisture, heat, light and aging. Unfortunately, most supplements are packaged with materials and technology that are so outdated and obsolete that they do little to protect product potency. These packaging materials only serve as a convenient container to hold and transport the product.

High bioactivity ingredients introduce a new problem. Not only are these ingredients highly active in your system, but they are also extremely active before you consume them. When a high bioactivity formula is exposed to air, moisture, light and heat, it can undergo chemical changes that damage its nutrients. In most cases, manufacturers do not include high bioactivity nutrients because of their expense. However, in the rare instances that they do, it is of little benefit unless they are protected by advanced packaging materials.

The high cost of these newly developed packaging materials accounts for their absence from popular supplements. There is little need to invest in costly materials to protect the inexpensive, low bioactivity ingredients and additives that dominate these formulas. Regrettably, these inexpensive products are generally found in unprotective containers or at best in cellophane packets that provide no effective barrier to light, moisture or oxygen. Not surprisingly, most manufacturers ignore the numerous advances in the areas of multiple layer packaging materials.

The Problem: *The Risks Of Product Tampering*

The Solution: *Tamper Proof, Laboratory Direct Products*

Product tampering is most easily eliminated by removing the product from contact with the public. It can also be prevented by packaging materials that provide tamper proof seals and then shipping this laboratory-sealed product directly to the consumer.

The Facts:

A capsule is the medically preferred form of consuming a nutritional supplement. Unfortunately, it is also the form most readily subjected to tampering. Over the past several years, there have been a number of instances of encapsulated retail shelf products being exposed to tampering. Therefore, safety demands that the benefits of a capsule are best enjoyed when the risks of exposure to tampering are eliminated.

The first step to eliminating tampering is to remove the exposed product from retail store shelves. This is even more effective when combined with multiple barrier packaging. Products that are individually boxed, bottled, shrink-wrapped and even separately packeted provide barriers and evidence of any tampering. This not only eliminates tampering, it also helps the product retain its potency better. These are a few of the many ways to make capsules entirely safe. Unfortunately, all these changes cost manufacturers more money than they choose to invest in your safety.

The result is that manufacturers produce supplements that offer little protection against the risk of product tampering. They endure long waits in warehouses or on retail shelves exposed to possible tampering or damage. It has already been demonstrated that capsules stand the highest risk of tampering, yet they are the only truly effective means of delivering a supplement's nutrients. Ultimately, safety can only be assured by shipping a tamper proof laboratory-sealed product directly to the consumer since there will be no opportunity to tamper with the product. Ideally, an effective encapsulated product is packeted, bottled, shrink-wrapped and boxed at the manufacturer's laboratory. It is this total laboratory sealing at its point of manufacture that makes a product absolutely safe and tamper resistant. The laboratory sealed product can then be shipped directly to the consumer with no middlemen along the way.

The Problem: *Spoiled, Overpriced Supplements*

The Solution: *Small Production, Manufacturer Direct Products*
Potency and effectiveness are assured by promptly shipping a newly manufactured product directly to the consumer. A recently manufactured product is more potent and effective than a product delayed for months or years on its journey to the consumer or manufactured in huge quantities and stored for months at the manufacturer's facility.

The Facts:
Nutritional supplements on store shelves are older than they appear. Lengthy delays in the shipping, warehousing, shelving and selling of popular supplements results in "aged" products reaching the retailer. Unlike a fine wine, aging should be discouraged with nutritional supplements. Their fragile nutrients spoil much like the nutrients in fresh fruits and vegetables. Incredibly, it

often requires a year or more for a supplement to reach the consumer following production. The frequent delays and unpredictable conditions at the manufacturer, distributors, shippers and warehouses reduce product potency. Moreover, the costs of numerous marketing steps and profit-taking middlemen dramatically increase the selling price of these conventional retail products.

Before a supplement is produced, the manufacturer sets out to locate the various raw materials. Most often they have been stored in a warehouse at the factory and are prepared and organized for the upcoming manufacture of the supplement. These raw materials can often sit at a large manufacturer's warehouse for months or years before being used. Next, the manufacturer blends the ingredients together. Hopefully all the ingredients are available at one time or completion of the blending will be delayed for days, weeks or months. Once the formula is blended, it can then be granulated and either tableted or encapsulated. This can occur quickly or once again require lengthy delays. The tablets or capsules that are produced can then be stored for days, weeks or months before they are bottled and packaged.

If and when the packaging is complete the product is then stored for days, weeks or months before it is shipped to a major health foods distributor. It is generally most cost-effective for a manufacturer to produce large volumes of product and thereby reduce the cost of that product. This means that even more time will pass while this larger inventory of product awaits shipment out of the manufacturer's warehouse. Eventually, it is shipped to distributors, where it is once again subjected to unpredictable delays before it is eventually shipped to a retailer or the retailer's warehouse. The product is then stored by the retailer in a central warehouse or in at retail location itself. Eventually, it spends its last days, weeks or months on the retail shelf. It isn't surprising that the average retail product in the average retail store is far, far older than you ever dreamed possible.

Adding insult to injury is the inflated retail price of these "aged," inexpensively produced formulas. Each of these steps along the marketing and distribution chain introduce a large number of individuals and businesses who expect compensation and profits for their services. As a result of the costs associated with marketing and distributing a conventional formula, its retail price will be greater than ten times its original manufactured cost. Conventional marketing and distribution produces not only stale products; but they are also ridiculously overpriced.

The End Result: *You Have Become An Informed Consumer*

Until now, supplement manufacturers have deprived you of your ability to make aware supplement decisions. By becoming an informed consumer, you have reacquired your freedom of choice. You will no longer be victimized by an industry dominated by hype and deceptive claims. Selecting a nutritional supplement will not continue to be a risky or arbitrary decision. Instead, the skills you now possess will permit you to make decisions based upon features that insure optimum effectiveness with absolute safety.

If you have additional questions that are not addressed in this edition of *Understanding Vitamin-Mineral Supplements*, call us toll free at 800-800-1200 or write to us at The Winning Combination, 1753 Cloverfield Boulevard, Santa Monica, California, 90404.